SEIZURES

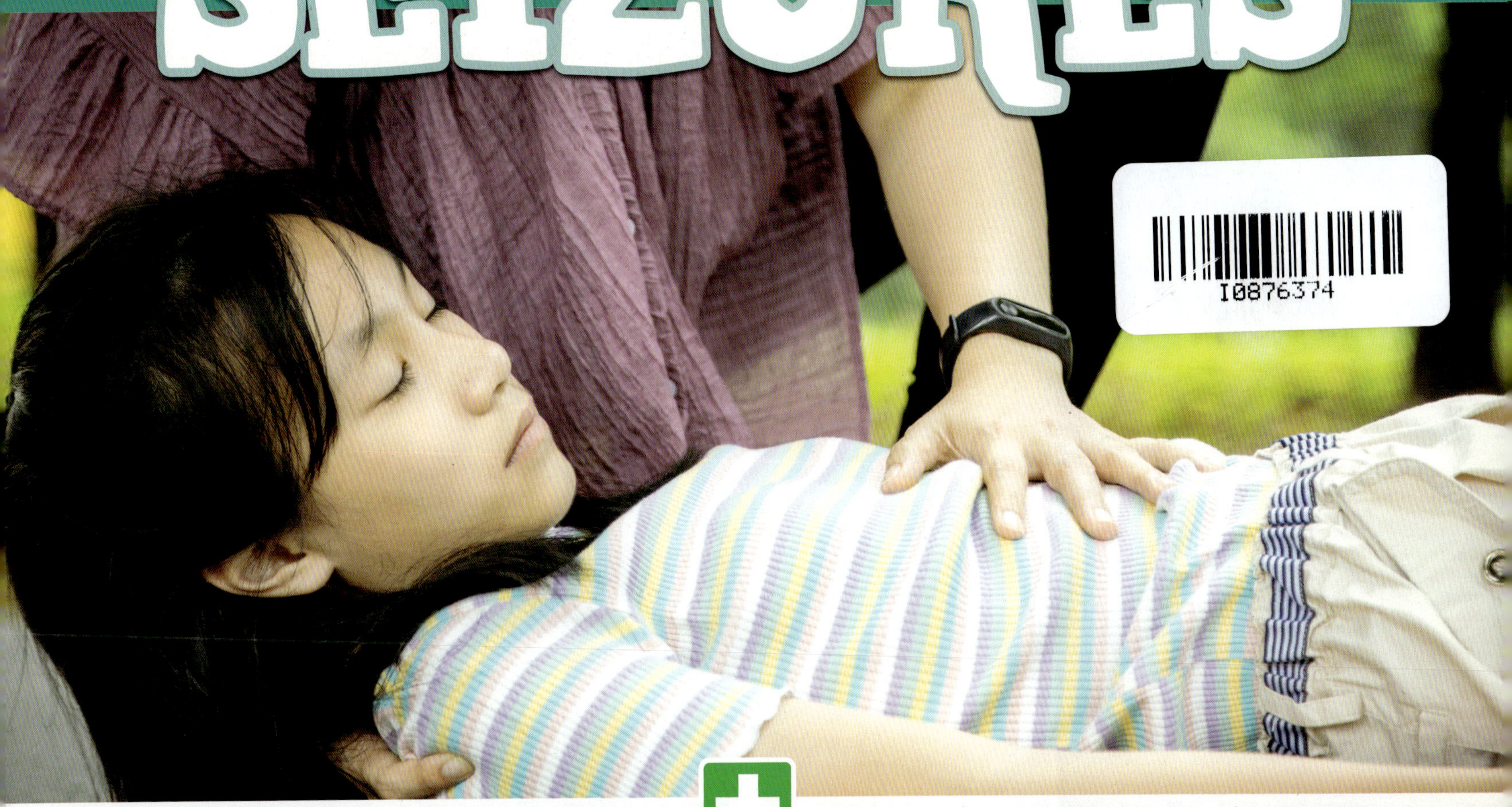

IN CASE OF EMERGENCY

Rochelle Groskreutz
and Ryan Smith

AV2
www.av2books.com

Step 1
Go to **www.av2books.com**

Step 2
Enter this unique code
EYJQWS91E

Step 3
Explore your interactive eBook!

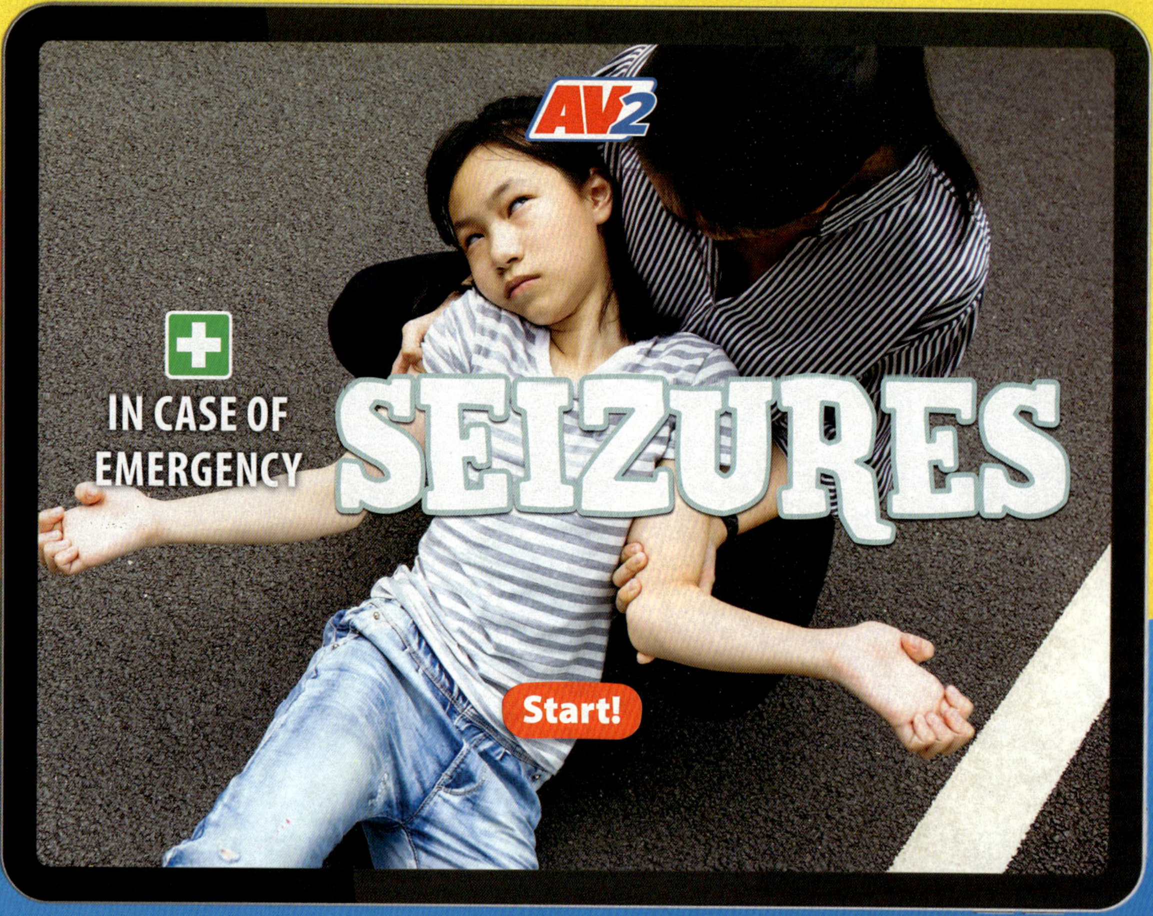

AV2 is optimized for use on any device

Your interactive eBook comes with...

Read

Audio
Listen to the entire book read aloud

Videos
Watch informative video clips

Weblinks
Gain additional information for research

Try This!
Complete activities and hands-on experiments

Key Words
Study vocabulary, and complete a matching word activity

Quizzes
Test your knowledge

Slideshows
View images and captions

View new titles and product videos at www.av2books.com

IN CASE OF EMERGENCY

SEIZURES

Contents

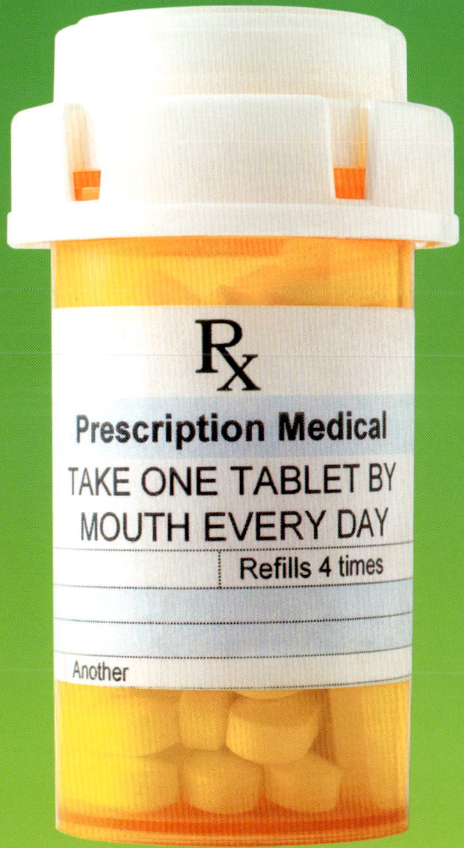

A Seizure

Some people have seizures.

Seizures can be caused by a head injury, a high fever, or epilepsy.

A seizure changes how a person feels and acts.

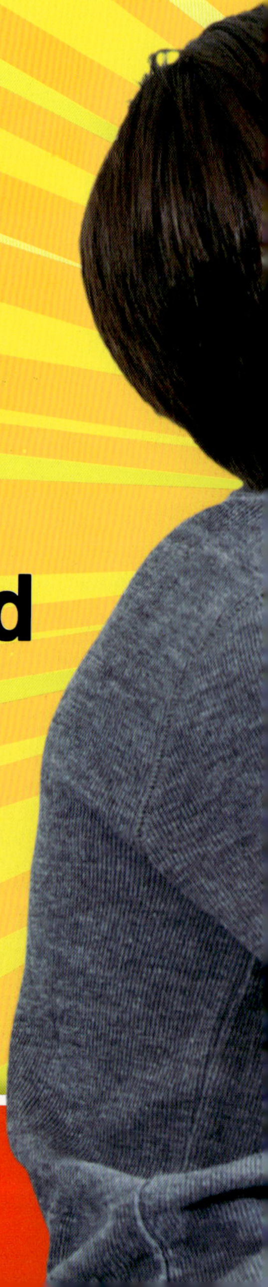

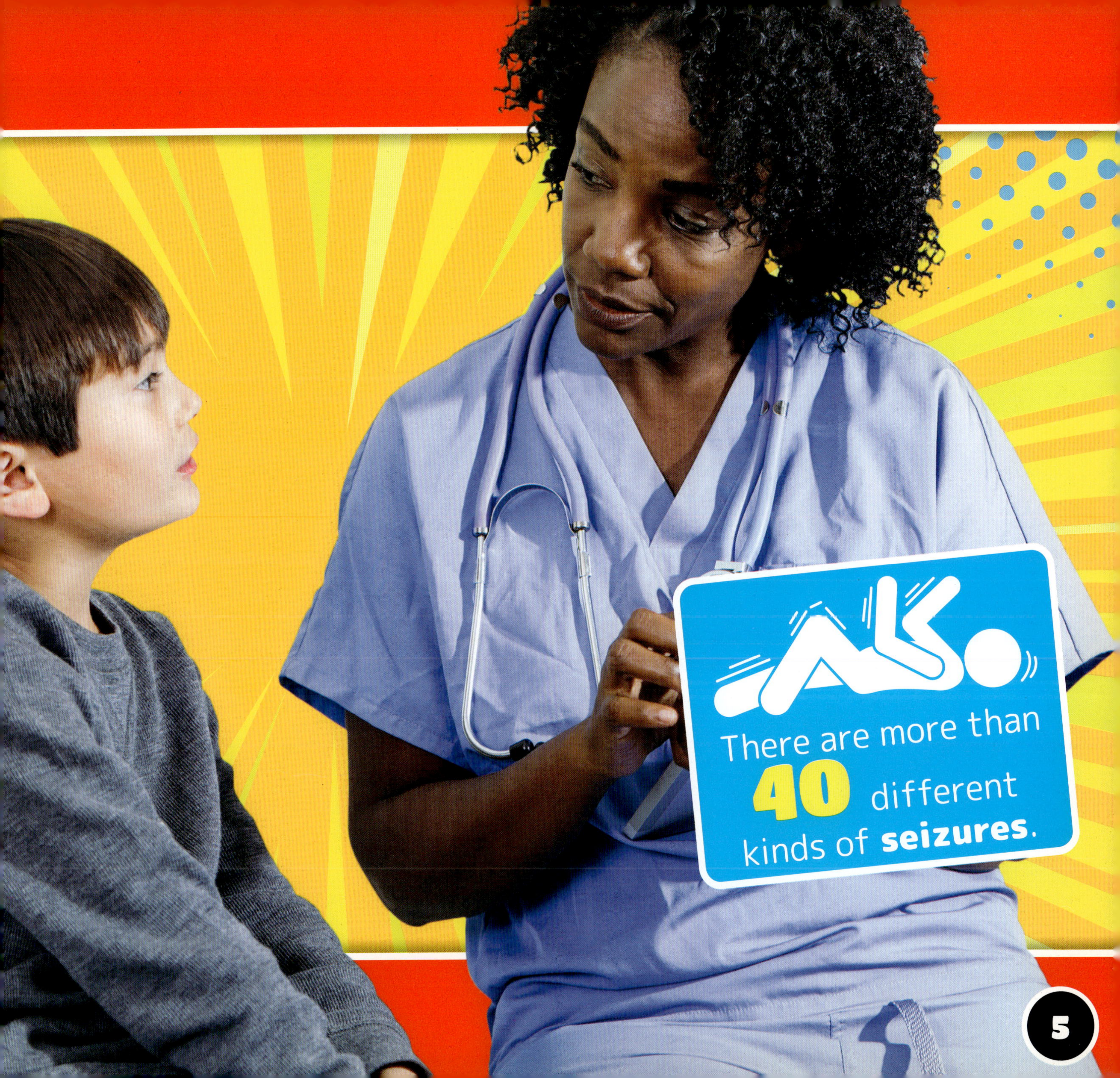

There are more than **40** different kinds of **seizures**.

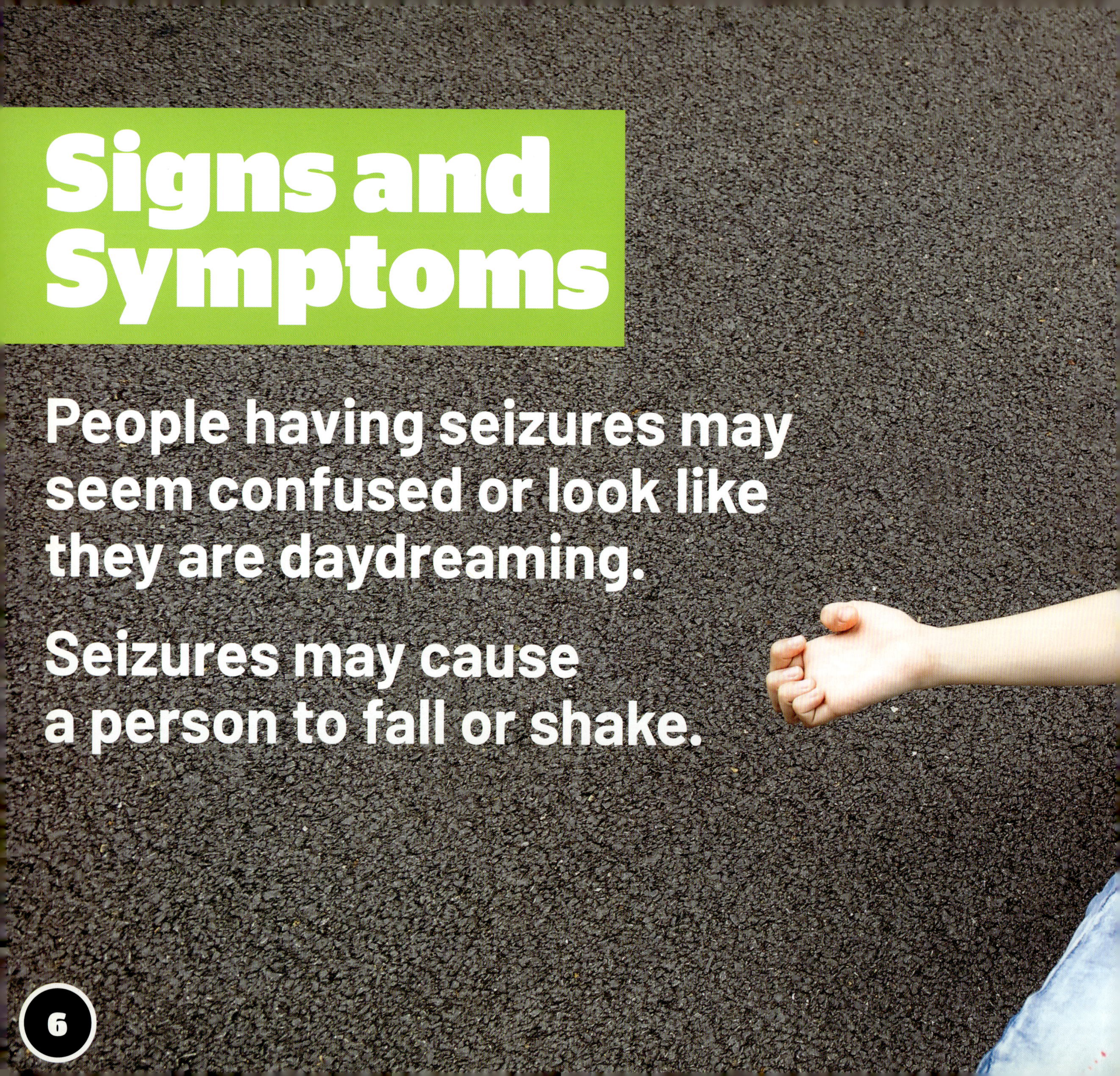

Signs and Symptoms

People having seizures may seem confused or look like they are daydreaming.

Seizures may cause a person to fall or shake.

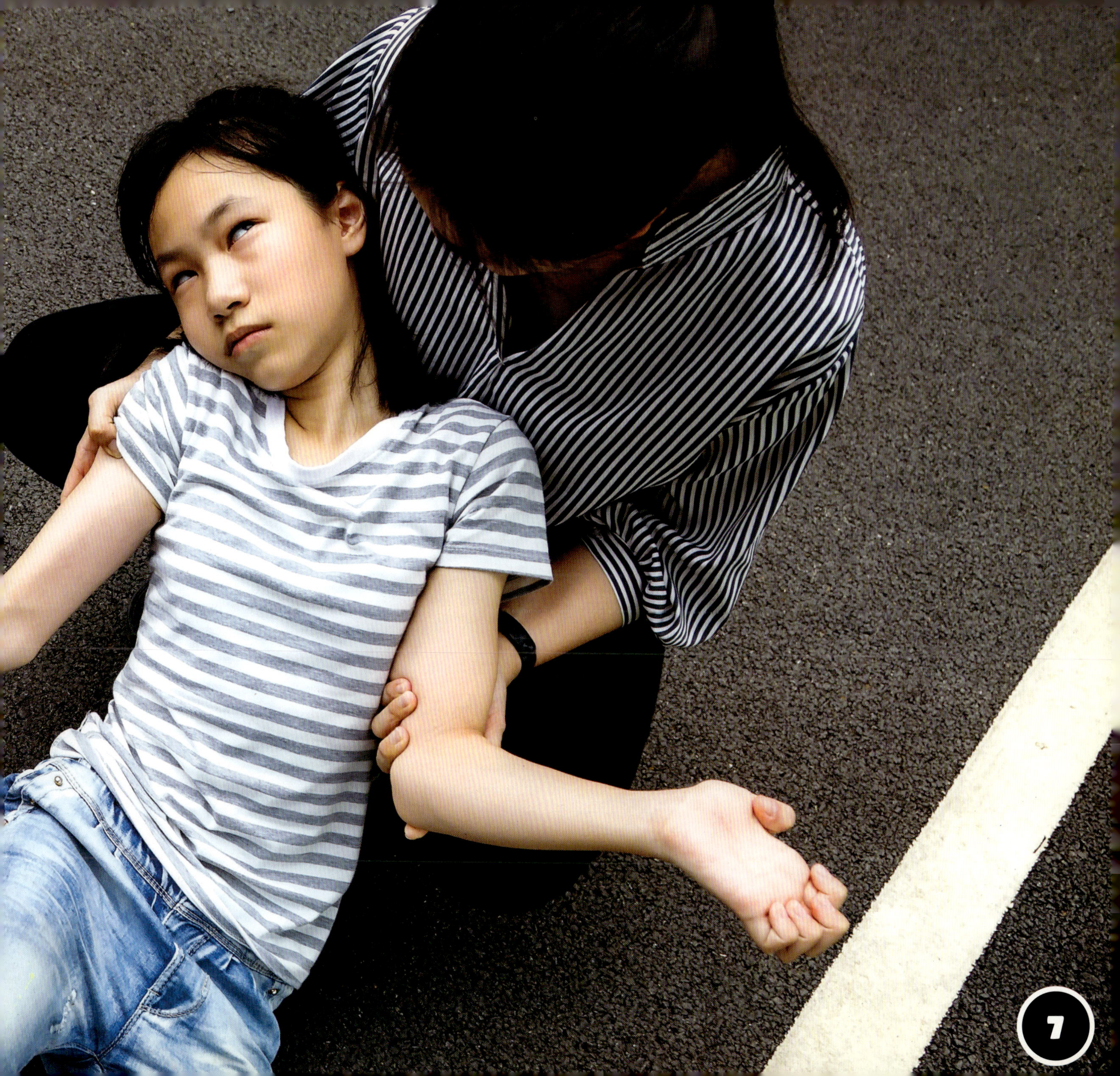

Stay Calm

It is important to stay calm when someone is having a seizure.

Keep yourself and others around you calm.

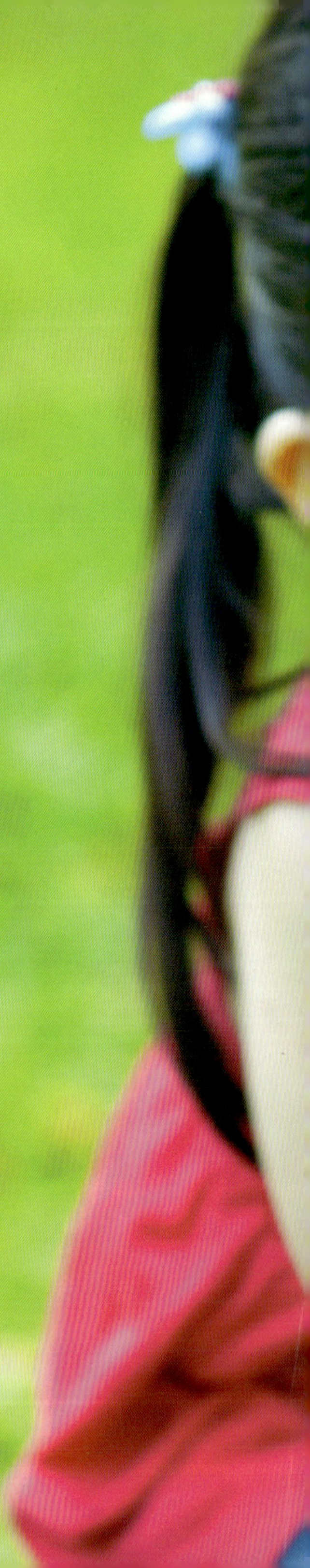

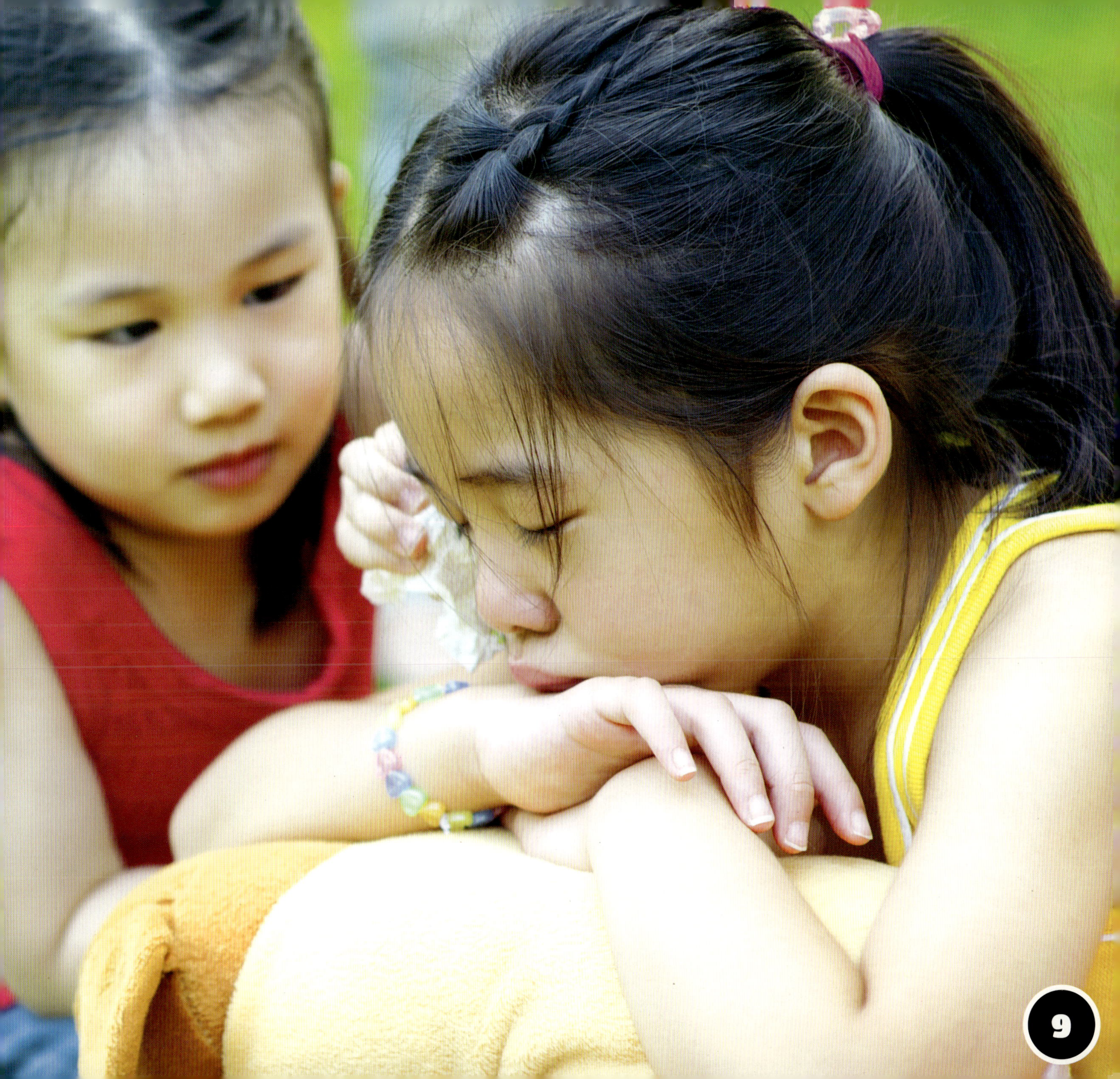

Call 9-1-1

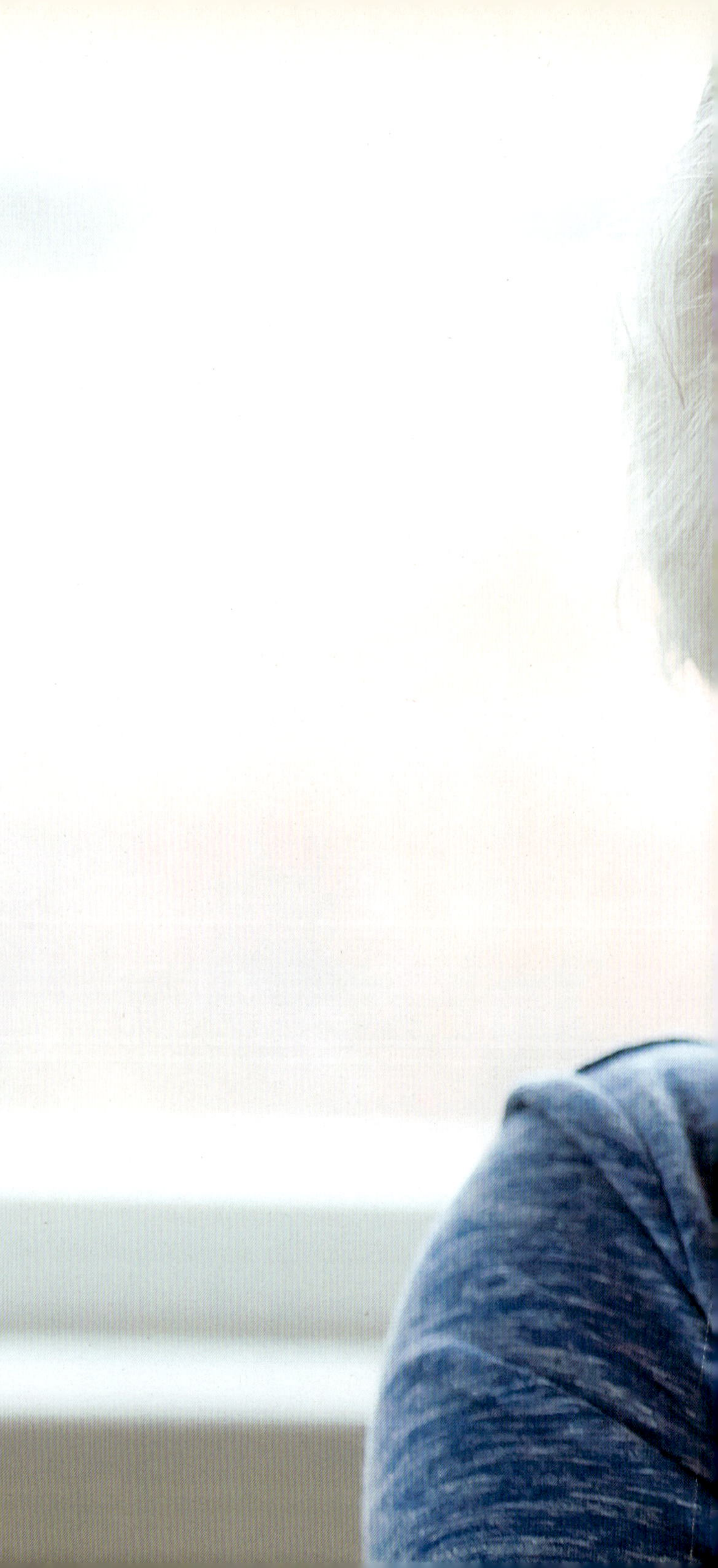

Call 9-1-1 if a seizure lasts longer than five minutes.

The 9-1-1 operator will need to know your name, where you are, and what the emergency is.

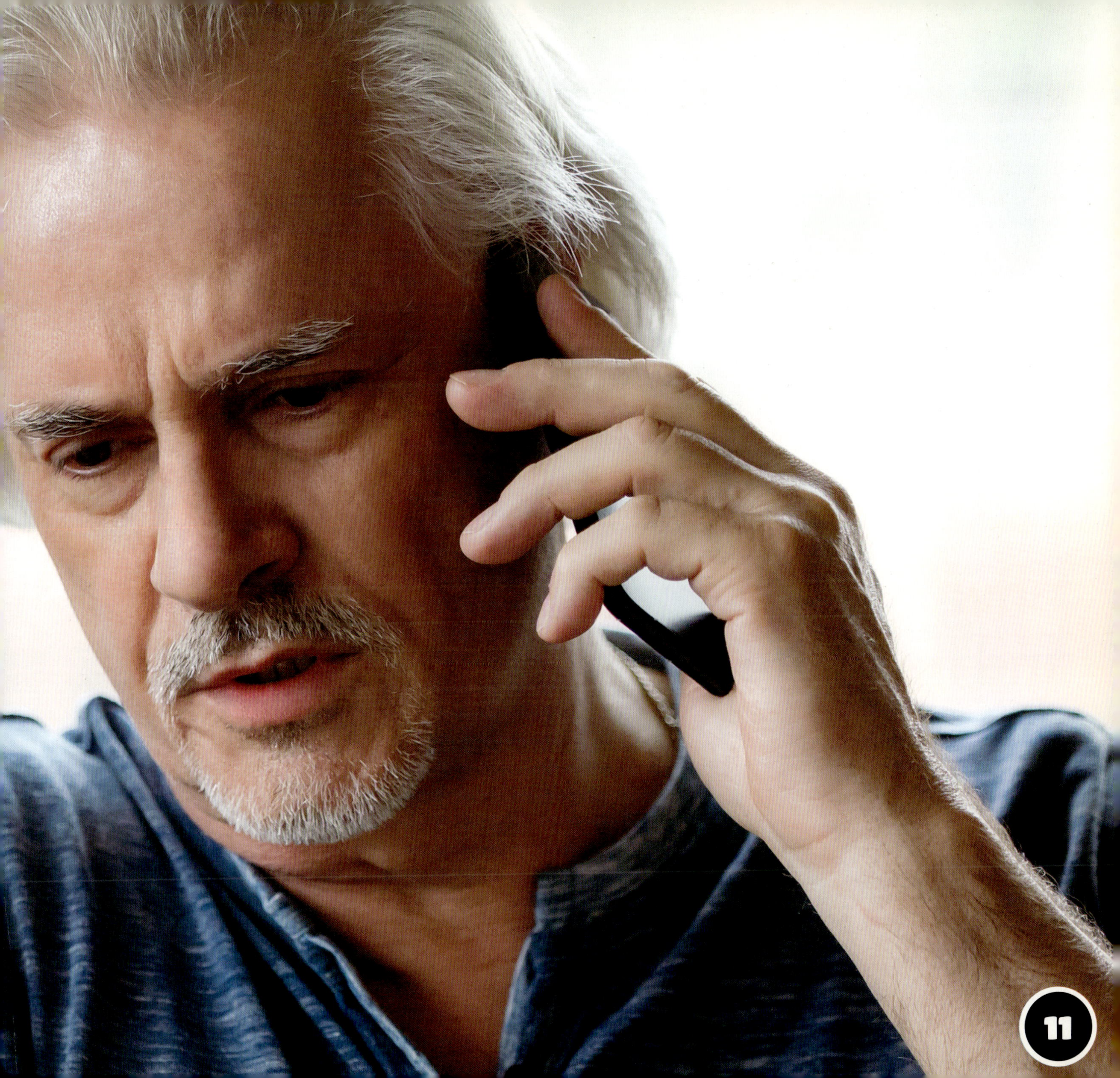

Clear a Space

Someone having a seizure can fall and get hurt.

Move objects out of the way and help the person lie down.

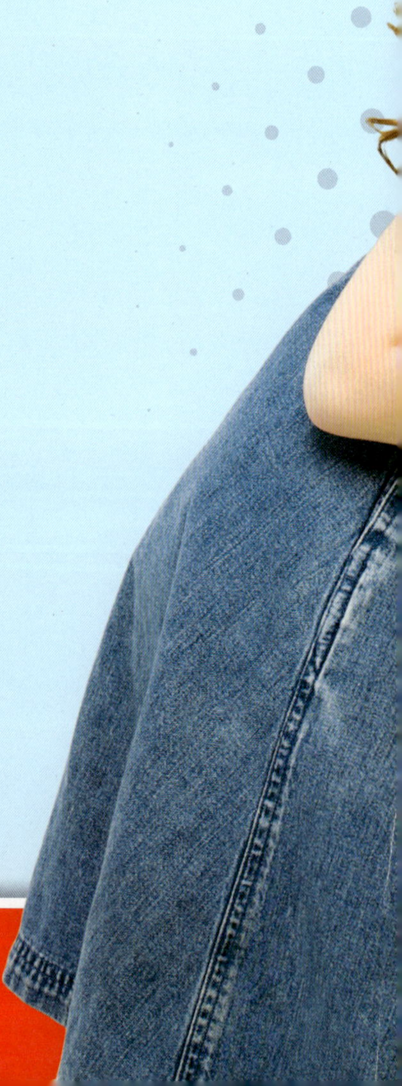

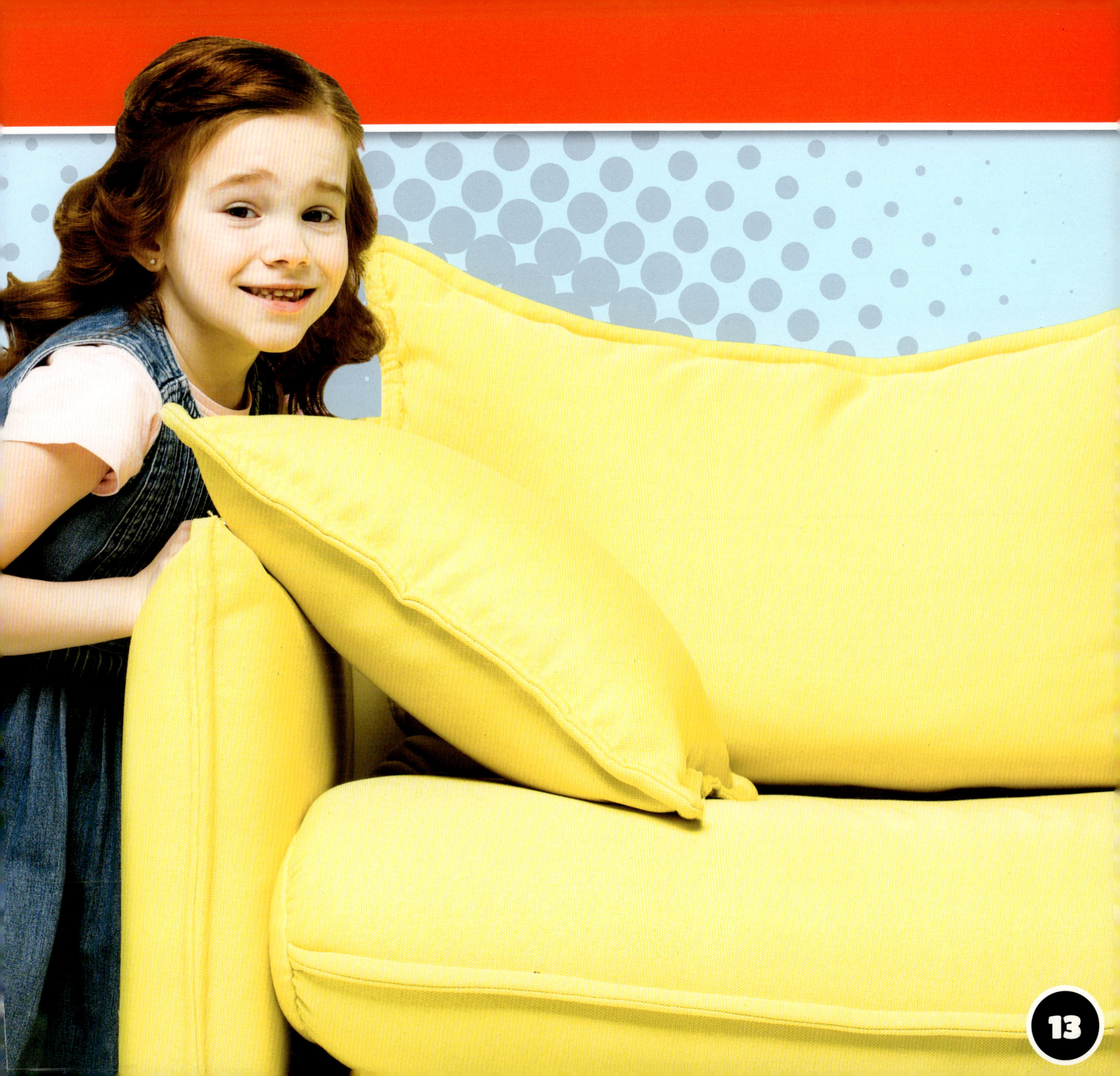

Stay with the Person

Put something soft under the person's head.

Do not try to stop the person from moving.

Stay with the person and wait for the seizure to end.

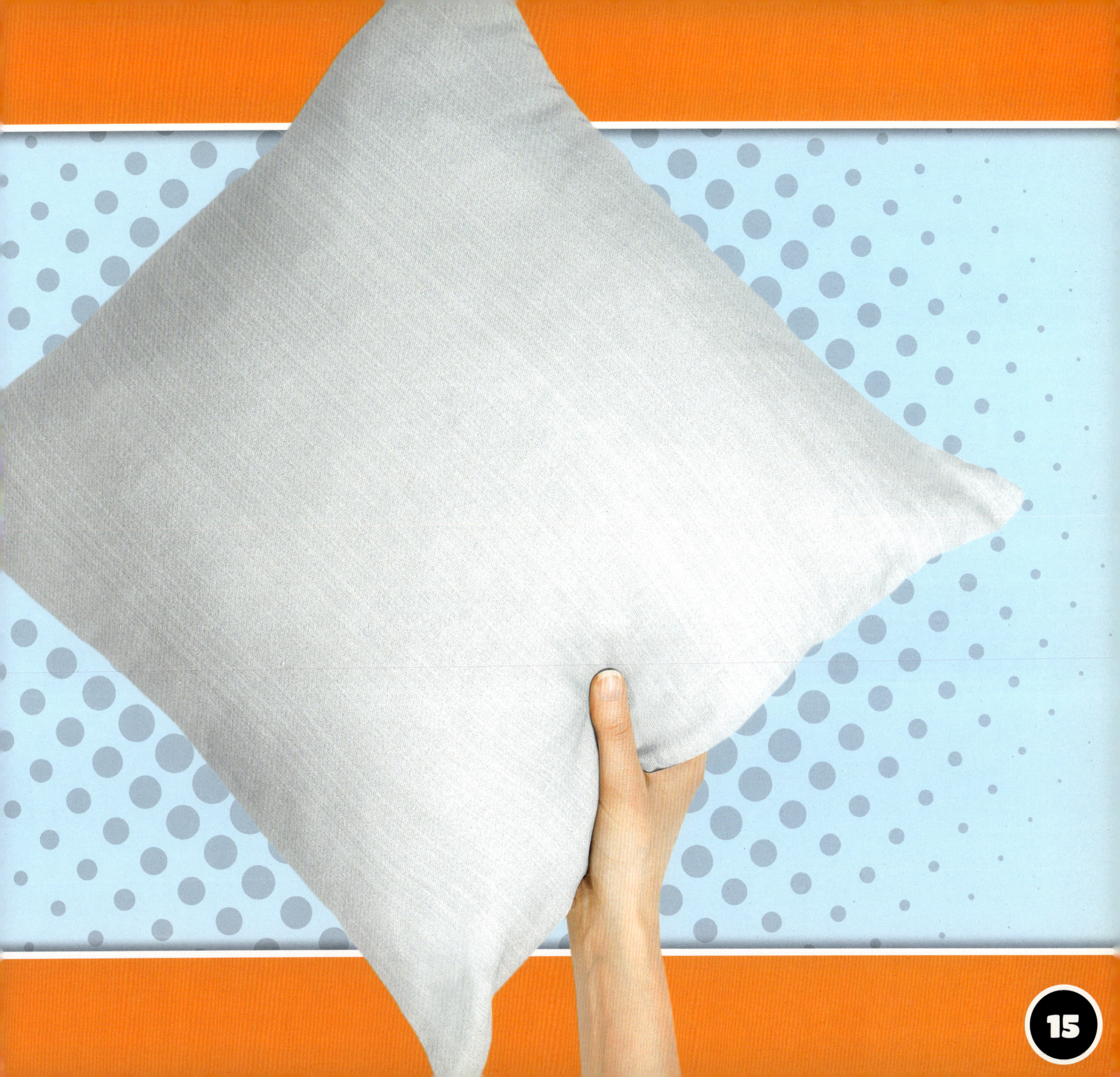

Rest

After the seizure, help the person sit down in a safe place.

Do not offer food or water until he or she is fully awake.

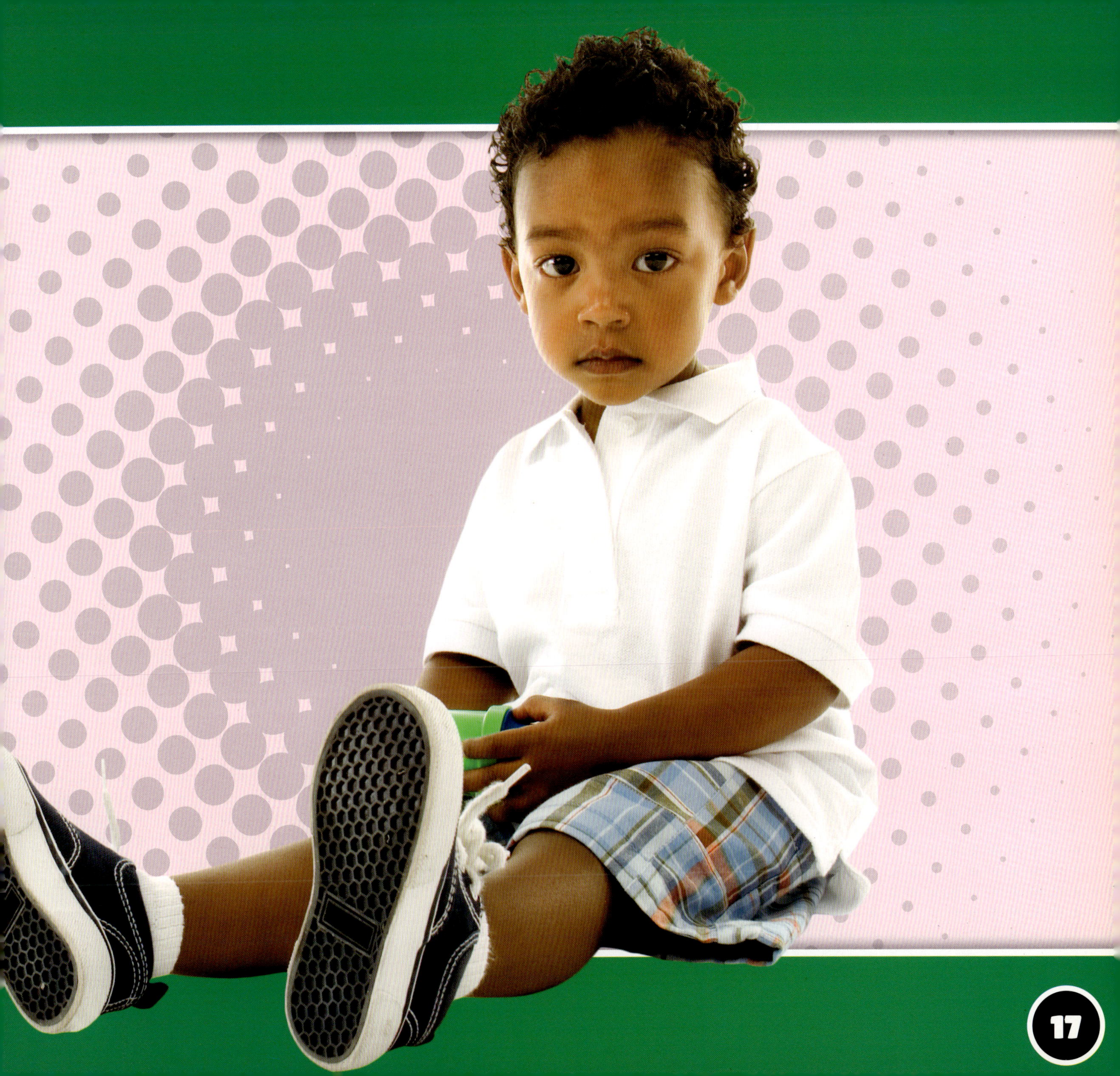

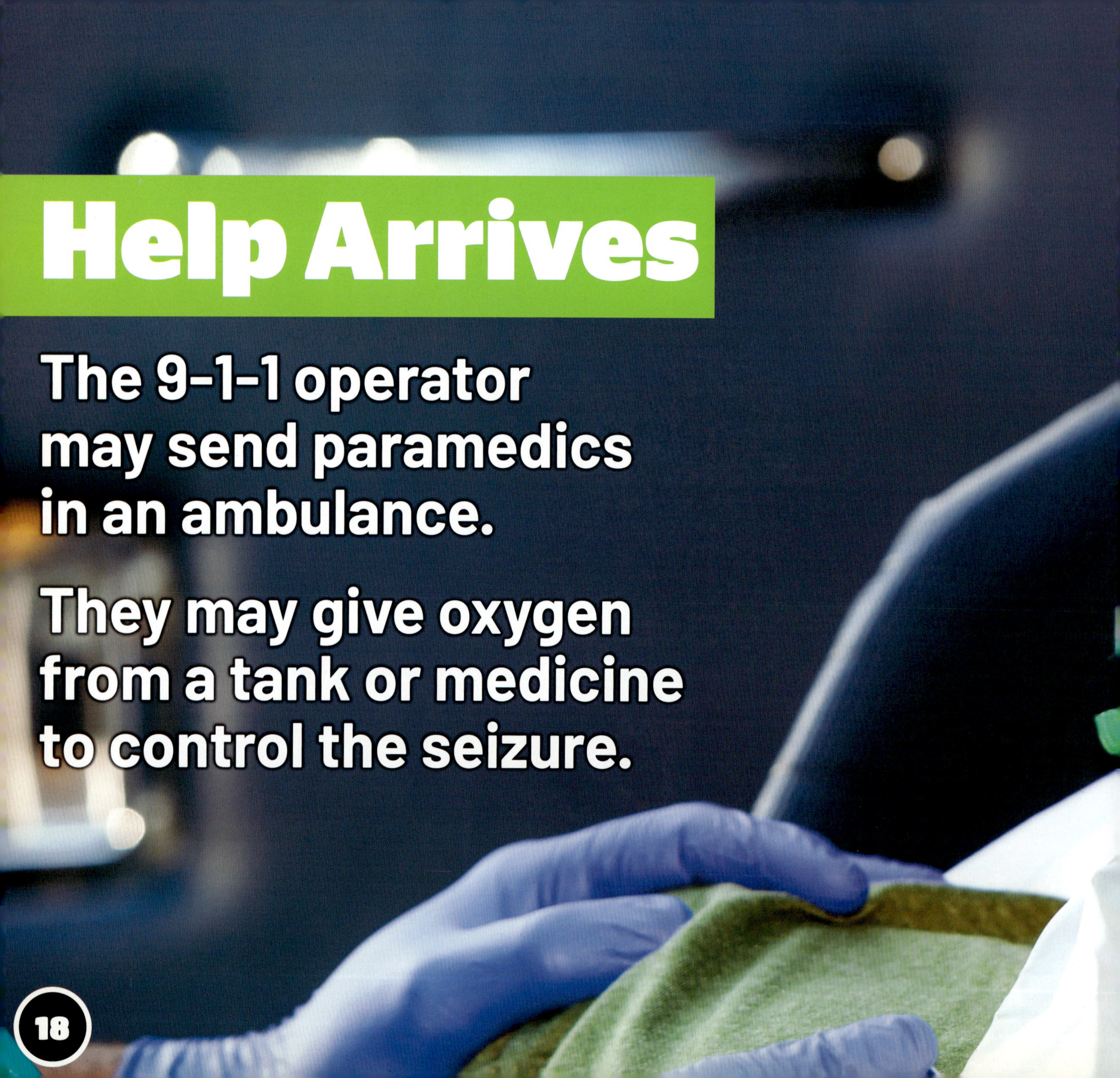

Help Arrives

The 9-1-1 operator may send paramedics in an ambulance.

They may give oxygen from a tank or medicine to control the seizure.

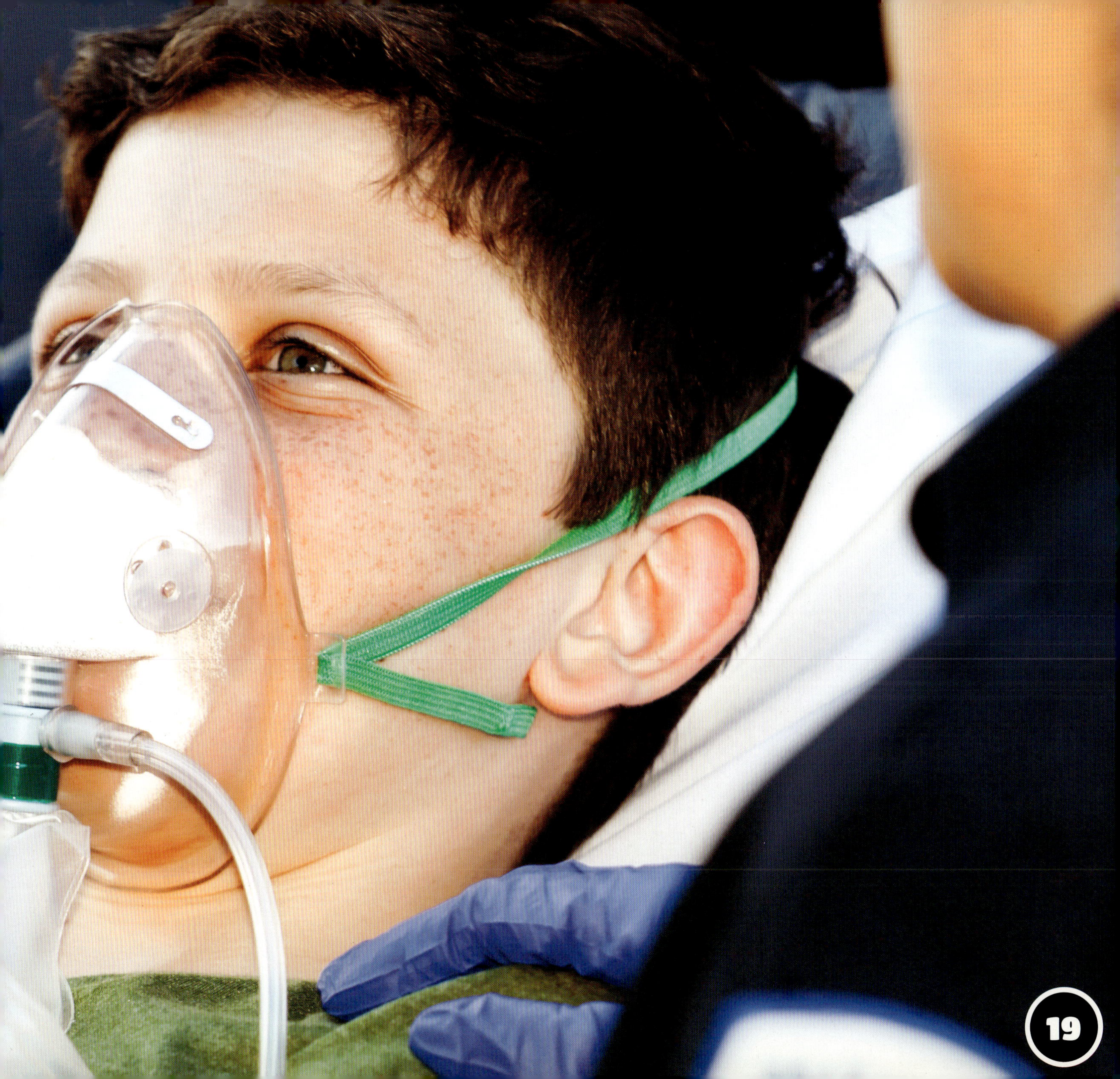

Preventative Measures

People who have seizures should get enough sleep, eat healthy food, and take their medicine.

They should also exercise and avoid flashing lights.

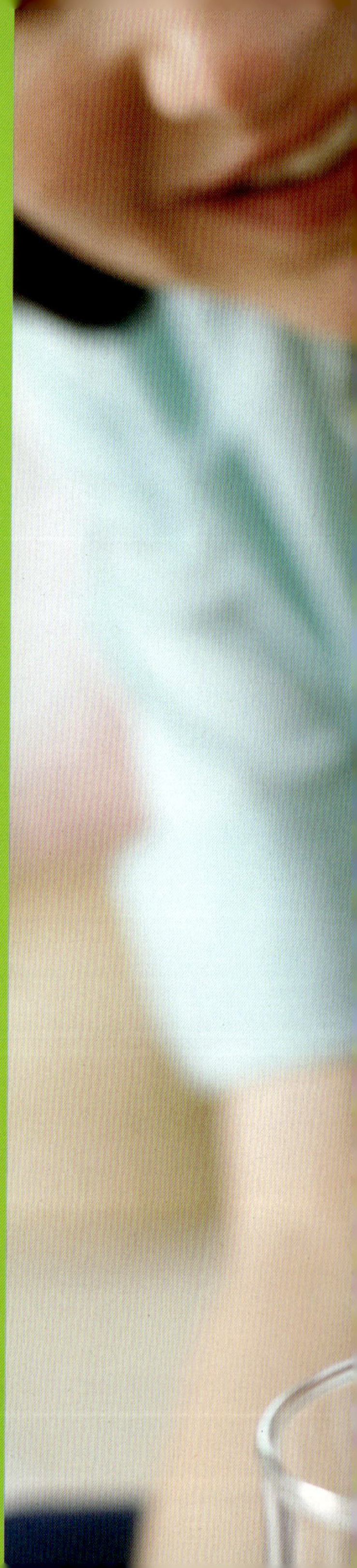

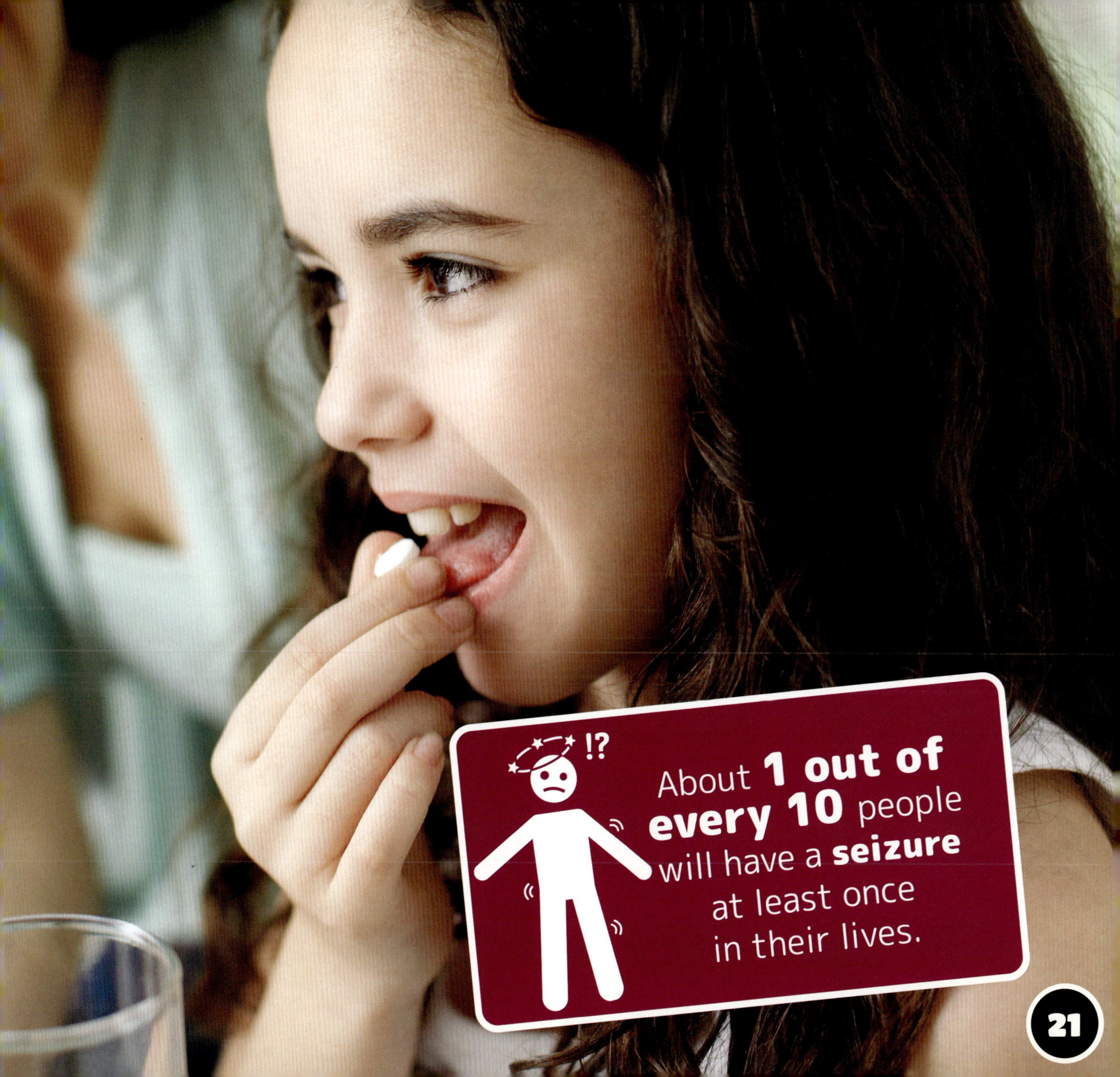

About **1 out of every 10** people will have a **seizure** at least once in their lives.

EMERGENCY PROCEDURES

These pages provide detailed information that expands on the emergency found in the book. They are intended to be used by adults as a learning support to help young readers understand the correct responses to each emergency featured in the *In Case of Emergency* series.

Pages 4–5

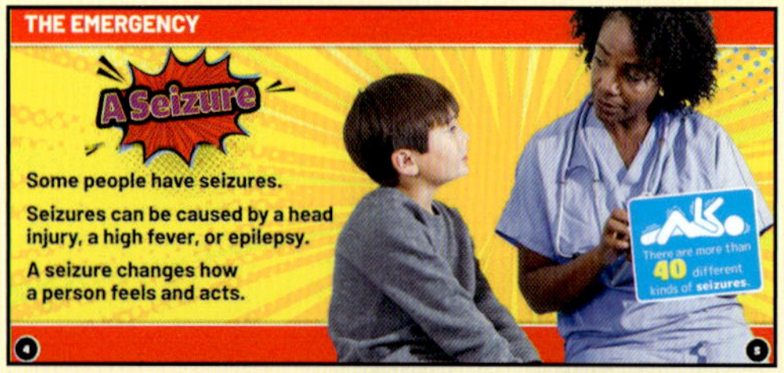

Some people have seizures. A seizure is a brief change in normal brain activity. Seizures are the main sign of epilepsy. Other conditions such as infections, high fevers, and head injuries can cause seizures, too. Seizures usually last from a few seconds to a few minutes. They can be triggered by factors such as lack of stress, a lack of sleep, or not taking seizure medication.

Pages 6–7

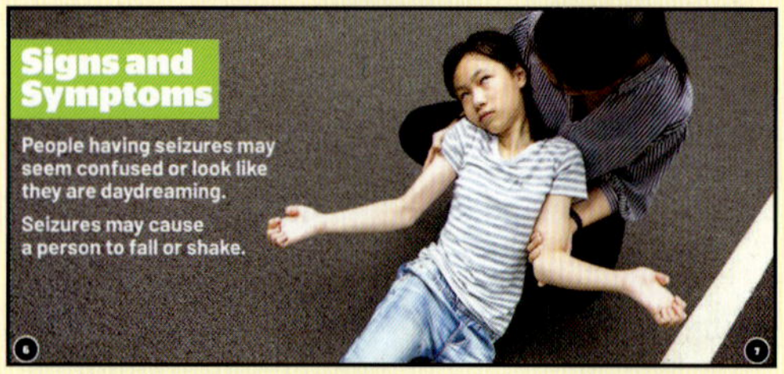

People having seizures may seem confused or look like they are daydreaming. There are many different kinds of seizures. Some seizures look like staring spells or cause small ticks such as lip smacking. Other seizures may cause a person to collapse, shake, and become unaware of his or her surroundings.

Pages 8–9

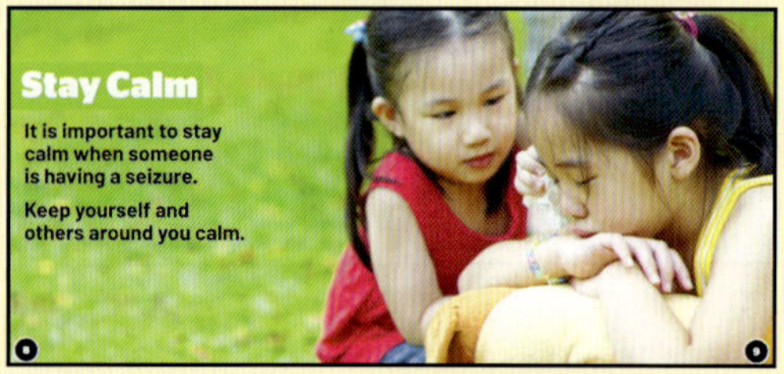

It is important to stay calm when someone is having a seizure. Remaining calm is important during any emergency situation. It is especially important for the person experiencing the seizure to stay safe and calm. Should the person start to panic, he or she may sustain self-injury or lose consciousness. Panicking bystanders may cause the person having the seizure to panic. The person helping must stay calm to avoid making any mistakes and to help the person having the seizure stay safe.

Pages 10–11

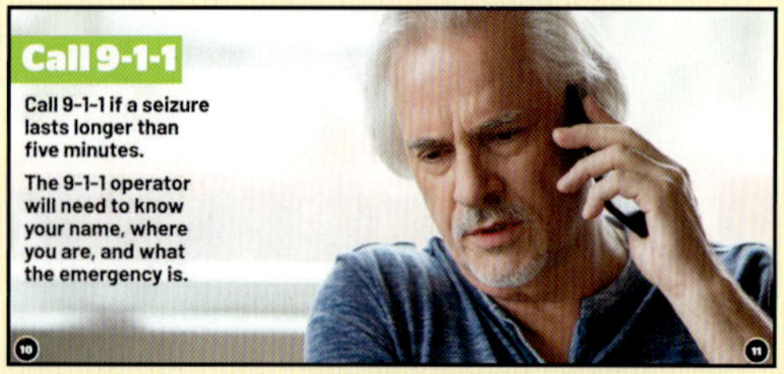

Call 9-1-1 if a seizure lasts longer than five minutes. A call to 9-1-1 should only be placed in emergency situations. Not all seizures are severe enough to warrant calling 9-1-1. Call 9-1-1 if a person has repeated seizures, passes out, or has difficulty breathing, or if the seizure lasts longer than five minutes. In less severe cases, a seizure can be treated without the assistance of paramedics or a doctor. 9-1-1 should also be called if the person has never had a seizure before, even if it is minor.

Pages 12–13

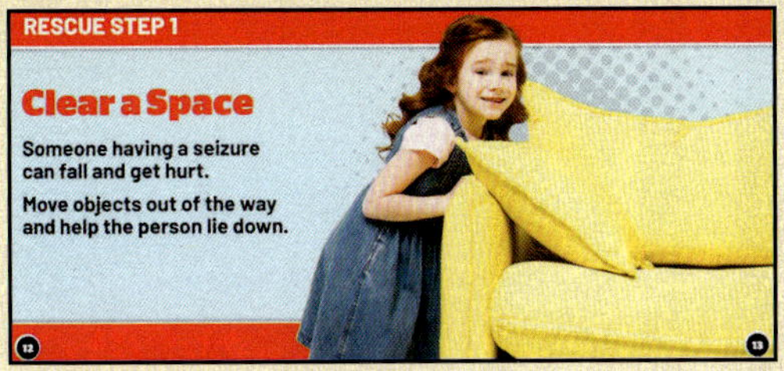

Someone having a seizure can fall and get hurt. The first step in treating a person having a seizure is to ensure that the person is in a safe space. Move any objects that the person could hit. Do not try to hold the person down or stop his or her movements during the seizure. Do not try to put anything between the person's teeth, either. He or she could have a spasm and bite down hard on the person offering treatment.

Pages 14–15

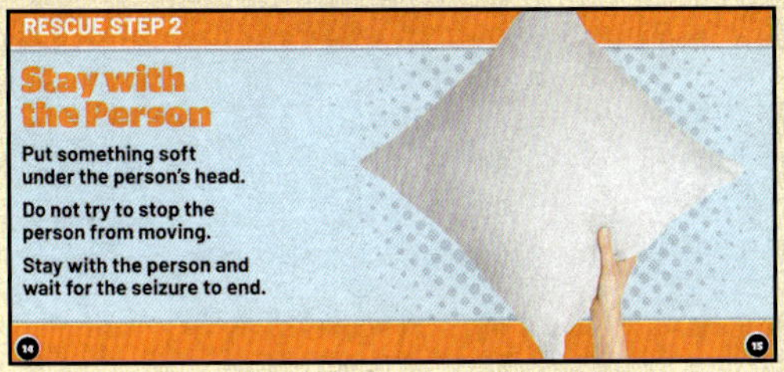

Put something soft under the person's head. Once the person is in a safe and comfortable space, remove glasses and loosen scarves, ties, or anything else that may make it hard for him or her to breathe. Help the person lie down and put something soft under his or her head. Time the seizure. Call 9-1-1 if it lasts longer than five minutes or if the person has multiple seizures.

Pages 16–17

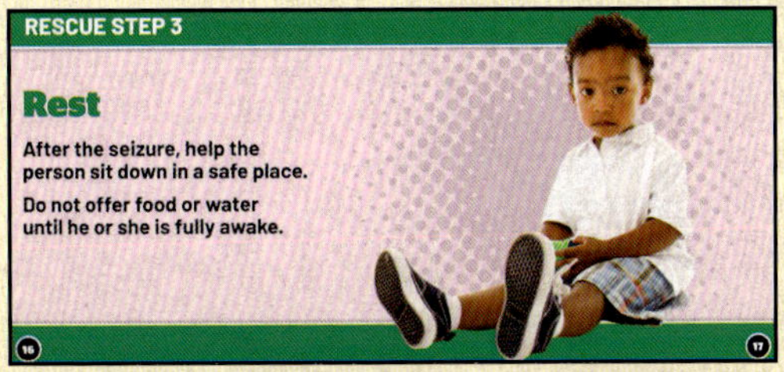

After the seizure, help the person sit down in a safe place. Sit with the person in a safe place once the seizure is over and provide comfort. Calmly explain what has happened. It is important to wait before offering the person any food or water. The food or water could become a choking hazard if the person passes out or has another seizure. If the person passes out, call 9-1-1. Lie the person down and ease the person onto his or her side with a hand under the cheek to help keep the airway open. Bend the person's top leg at the knee to prevent him or her from falling forward.

Pages 18–19

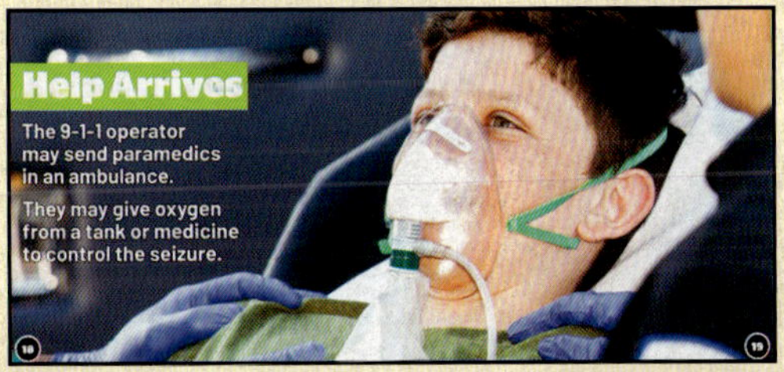

The 9-1-1 operator may send paramedics in an ambulance. Paramedics will assess the situation and monitor the person having the seizure. Paramedics are trained to provide oxygen from a tank to a person having a seizure. They are also trained to administer intravenous medicines that will help control the seizure. Even if the seizure seems to be over, paramedics will likely still take the person to the hospital to be monitored and evaluated by a doctor.

Pages 20–21

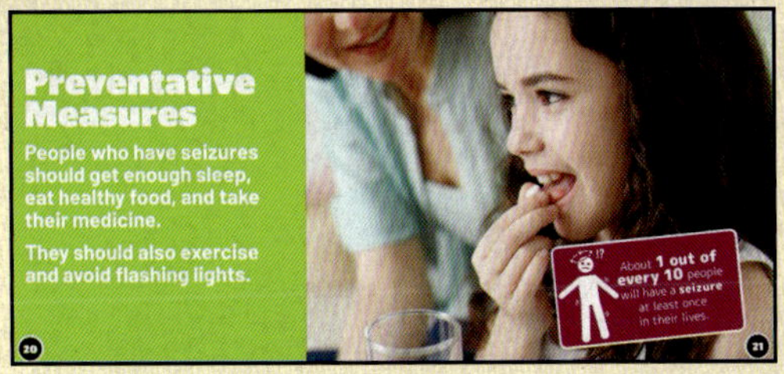

People who have seizures should get enough sleep, eat healthy food, and take their medicine. There is no cure for seizures, but they can be effectively controlled by medication that doctors prescribe. People who experience seizures must try to avoid situations, activities, or irritants that may trigger a seizure. Enough sleep, a healthy diet, and managing stress help prevent seizures. It also helps for people with seizure disorders to avoid bright, flashing lights and limit visual stimuli from video games, television, or computers.

KEY WORDS

Research has shown that as much as 65 percent of all written material published in English is made up of 300 words. These 300 words cannot be taught using pictures or learned by sounding them out. They must be recognized by sight. This book contains 85 common sight words to help young readers improve their reading fluency and comprehension. This book also teaches young readers several important content words, such as proper nouns. These words are paired with pictures to aid in learning and improve understanding.

Page	Sight Words First Appearance
4	a, and, be, by, can, changes, have, head, high, how, or, people, some, the
5	are, different, kinds, more, of, than, there
6	like, look, may, seem, they, to
8	around, important, is, it, keep, others, when, you
10	call, if, know, lasts, name, need, what, where, will, your
12	down, get, help, move, out, way
14	do, end, for, from, not, put, something, stop, try, under, with
16	after, food, he, in, place, she, until, water
18	an, give
20	also, eat, enough, lights, should, take, who
21	about, at, every, lives, once, their

Page	Content Words First Appearance
4	emergency, epilepsy, fever, injury, person, seizure
6	signs, symptoms
10	address, minutes, operator
12	objects, space, step
18	ambulance, medicine, oxygen, paramedic, tank
20	preventative measures, screen, sleep

Published by AV2
14 Penn Plaza 9th Floor New York, NY 10122
Website: www.av2books.com

Library of Congress Cataloging-in-Publication Data

Names: Groskreutz, Rochelle, author. | Smith, Ryan, author.
Title: Seizures / Rochelle Groskreutz and Ryan Smith.
Description: New York : AV2, [2021] | Series: In case of emergency | Audience: Ages 5-9 | Audience: Grades 2-3
Identifiers: LCCN 2020014492 (print) | LCCN 2020014493 (ebook) | ISBN 9781791126766 (library binding) | ISBN 9781791126773 (paperback) | ISBN 9781791126780 | ISBN 9781791126797
Subjects: LCSH: Spasms--Juvenile literature. | Medical emergencies--Juvenile literature.
Classification: LCC RC429 .G76 2021 (print) | LCC RC429 (ebook) | DDC 616.02/5--dc23
LC record available at https://lccn.loc.gov/2020014492
LC ebook record available at https://lccn.loc.gov/2020014493

Printed in Guangzhou, China
1 2 3 4 5 6 7 8 9 0 24 23 22 21 20

052020
100919

Project Coordinator: Ryan Smith
Art Director: Terry Paulhus

Every reasonable effort has been made to trace ownership and to obtain permission to reprint copyright material. The publisher would be pleased to have any errors or omissions brought to their attention so that they may be corrected in subsequent printings.

The publisher acknowledges iStock and Shutterstock as its primary image suppliers for this title.